Sirtfood Diet Mastery

Definitive Guide To Easy, Healthy, And Mouthwatering Recipes For A Rapid Weight Loss, A Meal Plan To Turn On Your Skinny Gene, Burn Fat, Boost Energy, And Reset Metabolism

Tanya Ross

Copyright – 2021 – All rights reserved.

The content contained within this book may not be reproduced, duplicated or transmitted without direct written permission from the author or the publisher.

Under no circumstances will any blame or legal responsibility be held against the publisher, or author, for any damages, reparation, or monetary loss due to the information contained within this book. Either directly or indirectly.

Legal Notice:

This book is copyright protected. This book is only for personal use. You cannot amend, distribute, sell, use, quote or paraphrase any part, or the content within this book, without the consent of the author or publisher.

Disclaimer Notice:

Please note the information contained within this document is for educational and entertainment purposes only. All effort has been executed to present accurate, up to date, and reliable, complete information. No warranties of any kind are declared or implied. Readers acknowledge that the author is not engaging in the rendering of legal, financial, medical or professional advice. The content within this book has been derived from various sources. Please consult a licensed professional before attempting any techniques outlined in this book.

By reading this document, the reader agrees that under no circumstances is the author responsible for any losses, direct or indirect, which are incurred as a result of the use of information contained within this document, including, but not limited to, - errors, omissions, or inaccuracies.

TABLE OF CONTENTS

INTRODUCTION **10**
MEAL PLAN **12**
Day 1: Monday **12**
Day 2: Tuesday **14**
Day 3: Wednesday **16**
Day 4: Thursday **18**
Day 5: Friday **20**
Day :6 Saturday **22**
Day 7: Sunday **24**
Breakfast Choices Recipes **26**
Twice Baked Breakfast Potatoes **26**
Sirt Muesli **29**
Beef Stroganoff French Bread Toast **31**
Classic French Toast **34**
Snack Recipes **36**
Chocolate Dipped Bananas **36**
Cinnamon Apple Chips **38**
Avocado Brownies **41**

Super Salads Recipes.......................... 44
Chicken & Kale Salad 44
Chicken & Berries Salad...................... 47
Chicken Salad 49
Soups and Broths Recipes 52
Lentil Soup 52
Spicy Pumpkin Soup 54
Speedy Suppers Recipes..................... 56
Kale and Turmeric Chicken Salad and Honey Lime Dressing 56
Turmeric Baked Salmon...................... 60
Buckwheat with Chicken, Kale and Miso Dressing 63
Main Meals Recipe 66
Strawberry Buckwheat Tabbouleh...... 66
Chili Con Carne 68
Spinach and Eggplant Casserole 71
Desserts Recipes 74
Green Tea and Vanilla Cream.............. 74
Figs Pie... 76
Chocolate and Chili Tart...................... 77

Beverage Recipes 80
Berry and Beet Smoothie 80
Irish Coffee 82
Double Melon Mojito 85
Dinner Recipes 88
Blue Cheese Pork Chops 88
Carnitas 90
Carnitas Nachos 92
Other Sirtfood Recipes 94
Turkey Breakfast Sausages 94
Banana and Blueberry Muffins 96
Morning Meal Sausage Gravy 98
CONCLUSION 100

INTRODUCTION

Thank you very much for purchasing this sirtfood cookbook. In this cookbook you will find a food plan designed especially for you and a series of recipes that you can make. The foods I am about to suggest are composed of surtine. There is a promise in consuming more Sirtfoods to activate the miraculous Sirtuins. The promise is in the evidence that Sirtfoods can help increase or decrease these human body functions and, along with other healthy lifestyle habits, will advantageously increase longevity and contribute to weight loss if these Sirtuins are activated. I really hope that my recipes and my meal plan can help you keep you young and fit, without making you feel the burden of too poor nutrition.
Enjoy.

MEAL PLAN

Day 1: Monday

Stir Fry Prawns with Kale and Buckwheat Noodles

3 Portions of Green Juice

Breakfast: Soy Yogurt with Mixed Berries, Chopped Walnut and Dark Chocolate.

Nutritional Value of Soy Yogurt with Mixed Berries per Serving: Calories 180, Fat 3.5 g, Cholesterol 0.0 mg, Sodium 25.0 mg, Potassium 48.0 mg, Total Carbohydrate 34.0 g, Protein 6.0 g.

Lunch: A Sirtfood Green Juice Salad Made with Kale, Celery, Apple, Parsley, Walnut Topped with Olive Oil Mixed with Lemon Juice and Ginger.

Nutritional Value of Sirtfood Green Juice Salad per Serving: Calories 557, Fat 17.0 g, Cholesterol 0.0 mg, Sodium 90.0 mg, Potassium 1,552.0 mg, Total Carbohydrate 96.0 g, Protein 11.0 g.

Snack: Celery and Hummus.

Nutritional Value of Celery and Hummus per Serving: Calories 122.6, Fat 6.1 g, Cholesterol 0.0 mg, Sodium 335.5 mg, Potassium 473.0 mg, Total Carbohydrate 12.6 g, Protein 5.7 g.

Dinner: Stir Fry Prawns with Kale and Buckwheat Noodles.

Nutritional Value of Stir Fry Prawns with Kale and Buckwheat Noodles Per Serving: Calories 208.0, Fat 39.1 g, Cholesterol 85.0 mg, Sodium 878.0 mg, Potassium 248.0 mg, Total Carbohydrate 59.2 g, Protein 58.0 g.

Day 2: Tuesday

Turmeric Baked Salmon

3 Portions of Green Juice

Breakfast: Mushroom Kale Omelette.

Nutritional Value of Mushroom Kale Omelette per Serving: Calories 187.7, Fat 13.5 g, Cholesterol 374.0 mg, Sodium 119.4 mg, Potassium 251.2 mg, Total Carbohydrate 4.3 g, Protein 12.3 g.

Lunch: Rocket Salad tuna, tomatoes and cucumber dressed in olive oil.

Nutritional Value Rocket Salad Tuna per Serving: Calories 337, Fat 54.0 g, Cholesterol 300.0 mg, Sodium 700.0 mg, Potassium 51.2 mg, Total Carbohydrate 5.3 g, Protein 10.5g.

Snack: Walnut.

Nutritional Value of Walnut per 100g Serving: Calories 654, Fat 65.0 g, Cholesterol 0.0 mg, Sodium 2.0 mg, Potassium 441.0 mg, Total Carbohydrate 14.0 g, Protein 15.0 g.

Dinner: Turmeric baked salmon.

Nutritional Value per Serving: Calories 205.3, Fat 14.0 g, Cholesterol 47.3 mg, Sodium 622.0 mg, Potassium 487.1 mg, Total Carbohydrate 2.0 g, Protein 17.6 g.

Day 3: Wednesday

Grilled Fish Buckwheat Salad

3 Portions of Green Juice

Breakfast: Fruit and Soymilk Smoothie.

Nutritional Value of Fruit and Soymilk Smoothie per Serving: Calories 171.1, Fat 3.1 g, Cholesterol 0.0 mg, Sodium 77.5 mg, Potassium 552.3 mg, Total Carbohydrate 32.8 g, Protein 5.5 g.

Lunch: Grilled Fish/Buckwheat Salad.

Nutritional Value of Grilled Fish/Buckwheat Salad per Serving: Calories 167.5, Fat 8.3 g, Cholesterol 55.5 mg, Sodium 624.3 mg, Potassium 454.9 mg, Total Carbohydrate 5.4 g, Protein 16.4 g.

Snack: Coffee.

Nutritional Value of Coffee per 8 Oz Serving: Calories 2.4, Fat 0.1 g, Cholesterol .0 mg, Sodium 4.7 mg, Total Carbohydrate 0.0 g, Protein 0.3 g, Caffeine 94.8 mg.

Dinner: Chicken and buckwheat noodles stir fry.

Nutritional Value of Chicken with Buckwheat Noodles per Serving: Calories 443.3, Fat 15.8 g, Cholesterol 68.4 mg, Sodium 3,741.7 mg, Potassium 532.4 mg, Total Carbohydrate 37.9 g, Protein 39.3 g.

Day 4: Thursday

Walnut

2 Portions of Green Juice

Breakfast: Muesli with Yogurt and Blueberries.

Nutritional Value of Muesli with Yogurt and Blueberries per Serving: Calories 280.2, Fat 3.5 g, Cholesterol 0.0 mg, Sodium 100.7 mg, Potassium 301.9 mg, Total Carbohydrate 57.4 g, Protein 10.9 g.

Lunch: Kale Salad with Edamame Beans and Red Onions Dressed in Olive Oil.

Nutritional Value of Kale Salad per Serving: Calories 84, Fat 7.3 g, Cholesterol 0.0 mg, Sodium 58.0 mg, Potassium 110.0 mg, Total Carbohydrate 3.9 g, Protein 1.2 g.

Snack: Walnut.

Nutritional Value of Walnut per 100g Serving: Calories 654, Fat 65.0 g, Cholesterol 0.0 mg, Sodium 2.0 mg, Potassium 441.0 mg, Total Carbohydrate 14.0 g, Protein 15.0 g.

Dinner: Tofu Burger with Whole Grain Bread and Salad.

Nutritional Value of Tofu Burger with Whole Grain Bread per Serving: Calories 220.0, Fat 4.5 g, Cholesterol 0.0 mg, Sodium 540.0 mg, Potassium 180.0 mg, Total Carbohydrate 27.0 g, Protein 16.0 g.

Day 5: Friday

Mushroom Kale Omelet

2 Portions of Green Juice

Breakfast: Mushroom Kale Omelette.

Nutritional Value of Mushroom Kale Omelette per Serving: Calories 187.7, Fat 13.5 g, Cholesterol 374.0 mg, Sodium 119.4 mg, Potassium 251.2 mg, Total Carbohydrate 4.3 g, Protein 12.3 g.

Lunch: Spicy Chicken Curry with Whole Grain Brown Rice.

Nutritional Value of Spicy Chicken Curry with Whole Grain Brown Rice per Serving: Calories 836.6, Fat 56.3 g, Cholesterol 20.8 mg, Sodium 76.0 mg, Potassium 648.6 mg, Total Carbohydrate 67.9 g, Protein 16.2 g.

Snack: Dark Chocolate.

Nutritional Value of Dark Chocolate per Serving: Calories 170.0, Fat 12.1 g, Cholesterol 1.0 mg, Sodium 6.0 mg, Potassium 203.0 mg, Total Carbohydrate 13.0 g, Protein 2.2 g

Dinner: Veggies Packed Spicy Tofu Stir Fry with Bird's Eye Chili.

Nutritional Value of Veggies Packed Spicy Tofu Stir Fry per Serving: Calories 189.0, Fat 8.0 g, Cholesterol 1.0 mg, Sodium 440.0 mg, Potassium 45.0 mg, Total Carbohydrate 18.0 g, Protein 12.0 g.

Day :6 Saturday

Coronation Chicken Salad

2 Portions of Green Juice

Breakfast: Braised Lentils.

Nutritional Value of Braised Lentils per Serving: Calories 215.0, Fat 5.3 g, Cholesterol 0.0 mg, Sodium 394.0 mg, Total Carbohydrate 295 g, Protein 14.3 g.

Lunch: Coronation Chicken Salad.

Nutritional Value of Coronation Chicken Salad per Serving: Calories 111.0, Fat 1.0 g, Cholesterol 41.0 mg, Sodium 798.0 mg, Total Carbohydrate 8 g, Protein 18.0 g.

Snack: Strawberries and Oranges.

Nutritional Value of Strawberries and Oranges per 200g Serving: Calories 110.0, Fat 0 g, Cholesterol 0.0 mg, Sodium 15.0 mg, Total Carbohydrate 8 g, Protein 1.0 g.

Dinner: Date and Walnut Porridge.

Nutritional Value of Date and Walnut Porridge per Serving: Calories 140.0, Fat 2.5 g, Cholesterol 0.0 mg, Sodium 190.0 mg, Total Carbohydrate 27.0 g, Protein 3.0 g.

Day 7: Sunday

Prawn Arrabbiata

2 Portions of Green Juice

Breakfast: Bun less Beef Burgers with All the Trimmings.

Nutritional Value of Bun less Beef Burgers with All the Trimmings per Serving: Calories 209.0, Fat 8.5 g, Cholesterol 57.3 mg, Sodium 658.0 mg, Total Carbohydrate 12.4 g, Protein 24.1 g.

Lunch: Smoked Salmon Omelette.

Nutritional Value of Smoked Salmon Omelette per Serving: Calories 288.1, Fat 9.2 g, Cholesterol 205.6 mg, Sodium 2,112.5 mg, Total Carbohydrate 15.6 g, Protein 33.1 g.

Snack: Celery and Hummus.

Nutritional Value of Celery and Hummus per Serving: Calories 122.6, Fat 6.1 g, Cholesterol 0.0 mg, Sodium 335.5 mg, Potassium 473.0 mg, Total Carbohydrate 12.6 g, Protein 5.7 g.

Dinner: Prawn Arrabiata.

Nutritional Value of Prawn Arrabbiata per Serving: Calories 500.6, Fat 12.4 g, Cholesterol 299.4 mg, Sodium 745.0mg, Potassium 671.2 mg, Total Carbohydrate 41.1g, Protein 48.8 g.

Breakfast Choices Recipes

Twice Baked Breakfast Potatoes

Preparation time: 1 hour 10 minutes.

Cooking time: 1 hour.

Servings: 2.

Ingredients:

- 2 medium reddish-brown potatoes, cleaned and pricked with a fork everywhere.
- 2 tablespoons unsalted spread.
- 3 tablespoons overwhelming cream.
- 4 rashers cooked bacon.
- 4 huge eggs.
- ½ cup destroyed cheddar.
- Daintily cut chives.
- Salt and pepper to taste.

Directions:

Preheat grill to 400°F.

Spot potatoes straightforwardly on stove rack in the focal point of the grill and prepare for 30 to 45 min.

Evacuate and permit potatoes to cool for around 15 minutes.

Cut every potato down the middle longwise and burrow every half out, scooping the potato substance into a blending bowl.

Gather margarine and cream to the potato and pound into a single unit until smooth— season with salt and pepper and mix.

Spread a portion of the potato blend into the base of each emptied potato skin and sprinkle with one tablespoon cheddar (you may make them remain pounded potato left to snack on).

Add one rasher bacon to every half and top with a raw egg.

Spot potatoes onto a heating sheet and come back to the appliance.

Lower broiler temperature to 375°F and heat potatoes until egg whites simply set and yolks are as yet runny.

Top every potato with a sprinkle of the rest of the cheddar, season with salt and pepper and finish with cut chives.

Nutrition:

Calories 647.

Fat 55.79g.

Carbs 7.45g.

Protein 30.46g.

Sirt Muesli

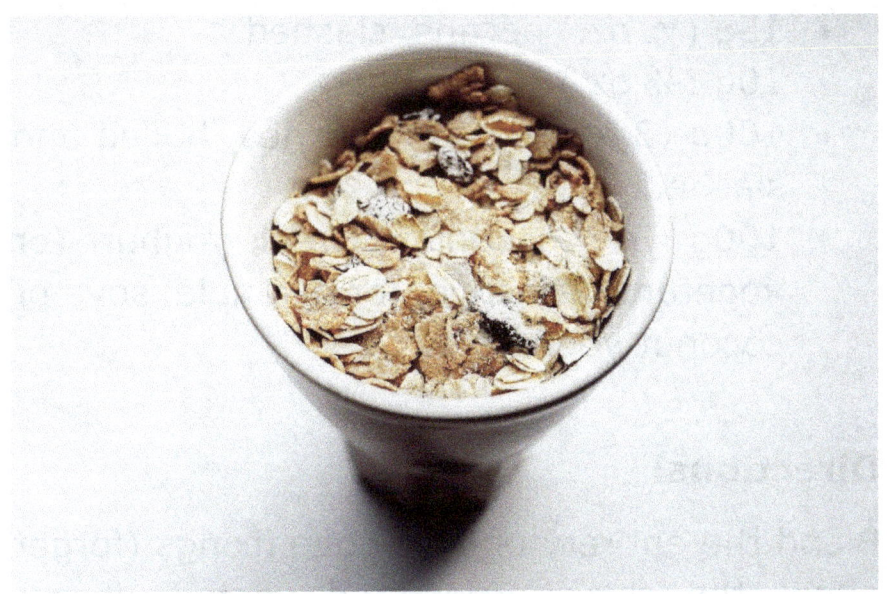

Preparation time: 30 minutes.

Cooking time: 0 minutes.

Servings: 2.

Ingredients:

- 20g (¾ oz.) buckwheat drops.
- 10g (⅜ oz.) Buckwheat puffs.
- 15g (½ oz.) coconut drops or dried up coconut.

- 40g (1 ½ oz.) Medjool dates, hollowed and slashed.
- 15g (½ oz.) pecans, slashed.
- 10g (⅜ oz.) cocoa nibs.
- 100g (3 ½ oz.) strawberries, hulled and slashed.
- 100g (3 ½ oz.) plain Greek yoghurt (or vegetarian elective, for example, soya or coconut yoghurt).

Directions:

Blend the entirety of the above fixings (forget about the strawberries and yoghurt if not serving straight away).

Nutrition:

Calories: 334.

Fat: 22.58g.

Carbs: 34.35g.

Protein: 4.39g.

Beef Stroganoff French Bread Toast

Preparation time: 10 minutes.

Cooking time: 15 minutes.

Servings: 2.

Ingredients:

- 4 tablespoons olive oil.
- 1/2 cups mushrooms.
- 2 teaspoons salt, separated.
- 1/2 teaspoon dark pepper.
- 2 tablespoons thyme.
- 2 tablespoons spread.
- 1/2 cup onions, diced.
- 2 cloves garlic, minced.
- 1-pound ground meat.
- 3 tablespoons generally useful flour.
- 2 teaspoons paprika.
- 1/2 cups meat juices.
- 1/2 cup sharp cream.
- 1 teaspoon Dijon mustard.

For the toasts:

- 1 portion French bread, inner parts dugout.
- 2 cups mozzarella.
- 3 tablespoons cleaved Italian parsley.

Directions:

Preheat stove to 350 degrees, and line a sheet container with material paper. Make the stroganoff: In a large Dutch grill or skillet, heat olive oil over medium warmth. Saute mushrooms with one teaspoon salt and dark pepper. Include thyme. Cook mushrooms until brilliant, roughly 4 minutes. Expel from a dish and put in a safe spot. Include margarine, onions and garlic to the container and saute 2 minutes. Cook ground hamburger over medium warmth until dark-coloured, roughly 4 minutes. Add flour and paprika to cover uniformly. Include meat soup, sour cream and mustard. Blend entirely and include mushrooms back in round the emptied portion with stroganoff and top with mozzarella cheddar. Spot on the readied heating sheet, and prepare for 5 to 10 minutes until cheddar is brilliant and softened. Head with parsley, cut and serve right away.

Nutrition:

Calories: 1007 kcal.

Protein: 88.04 g.

Fat: 60 g.

Carbohydrates: 32.06 g.

Classic French Toast

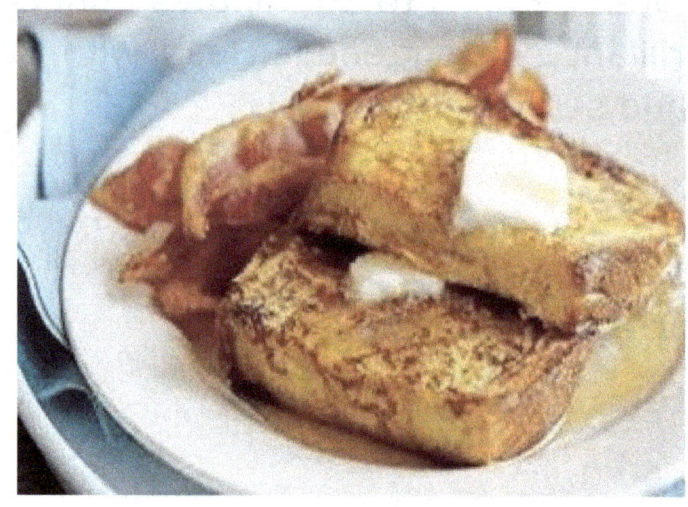

Preparation time: 10 minutes.

Cooking time: 45 minutes.

Servings: 2.

Ingredients:

- Four huge eggs.
- 1/2 cup entire milk.
- One teaspoon vanilla concentrate.
- 1/2 teaspoons ground cinnamon partitioned.
- 8 cuts Brioche bread.

Directions:

On the off chance that is utilizing an electric iron, preheat the frying pan to 350ºF.

Race until very much consolidated.

Plunge each side of the bread in the egg blend. Note - include the other portion of the cinnamon after you have plunged half of your bread cuts and blend once more. This will ensure the entirety of the cuts gets a decent measure of cinnamon.

Soften a little margarine on the hot frying pan or in a large skillet over medium warmth.

Serve the French toast warm with maple syrup, powdered sugar, and berries, whenever wanted.

Note - to keeps the French toast warm, heat the stove to 200ºF. Spot a wire rack on a massive preparing sheet and spot the French toast on the shelf. Keep warm in the grill for as long as 30 minutes.

Nutrition:

Calories: 110. **Carbs:** 26.5g.

Fat: 11g. **Protein:** 2.5g

Snack Recipes

Chocolate Dipped Bananas

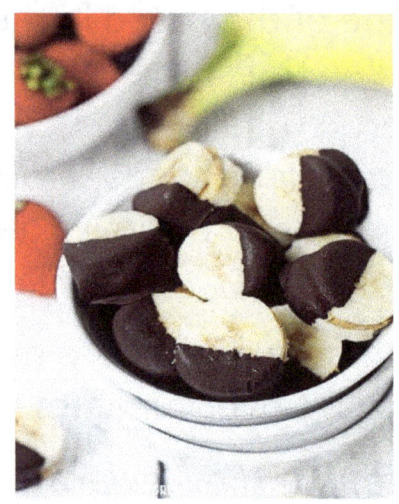

Preparation Time: 5 minutes.

Cooking Time: 0 minutes.

Servings: 9.

Ingredients:

- Dark chocolate – 12 Ounces.
- Bananas – 1 Large cut into thirds.
- Coconut oil – 1 Tbsp.
- Chopped, salted pistachios.
- Chopped, smoked almonds.

- Cocoa nibs.
- Popsicle sticks.

Directions:

In a double boiler, melt together the chocolate and coconut oil, stirring until smooth.

Use a silicone pad to cover a cookie pan and put to the side until needed.

Into one end of each banana, insert a Popsicle stick and dip the bananas into the chocolate, lightly tapping them on the side of the pot to remove excess.

Lay the bananas out onto the parchment and sprinkle with the chopped nuts and cocoa nibs.

Place in the baking sheet in the freezer to allow the bananas to harden and set.

Once fully frozen, serve or wrap individually to store in the freezer.

Nutrition:

Calories: 331.

Fat: 15g.

Carbs 48g.

Protein: 5.5g.

Cinnamon Apple Chips

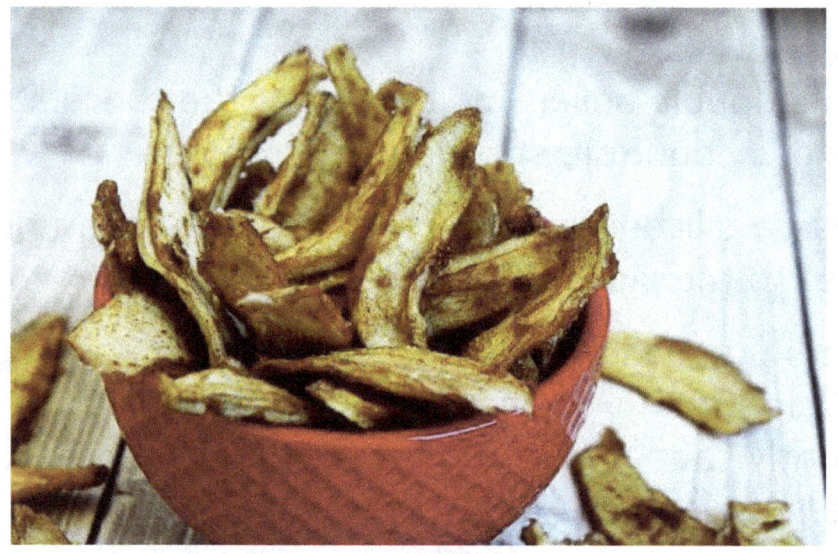

Preparation Time: 10 minutes.

Cooking Time: 2 hours.

Servings: 6.

Ingredients:

- Fuji apples – 3 larges.
- Ground cinnamon– .75 Tsp.

Directions:

Place your oven racks in the upper and lower portions of the oven and set to 200°F.

Cover 2 cookie sheets with silicone pads then put to the side until needed.

Wash the apples then remove the cores using an apple corer.

Using a mandolin, slice the apples to 1/8" thick slices.

Lay the apples out over the baking sheets and an even, single layer.

Sprinkle the apples with cinnamon and bake each pan on an upper and lower rack for 60 minutes.

After the 1 hour, take the pans and switch racks to move the pan that was on the upper rack to the lower and the one that was on the lower rack to the upper.

Continue to bake for 1-1/2 hours.

Test the doneness by removing 1 chip from a pan and letting it cool outside the oven for 2 - 3 minutes. If it is crispy after cooling, it is done.

Turn the oven off but let the apples stay in there for another hour to allow to cool and crisp.

Nutrition:

Calories: 220.

Fat: 0g.

Carbs: 13g.

Protein: 0g.

Avocado Brownies

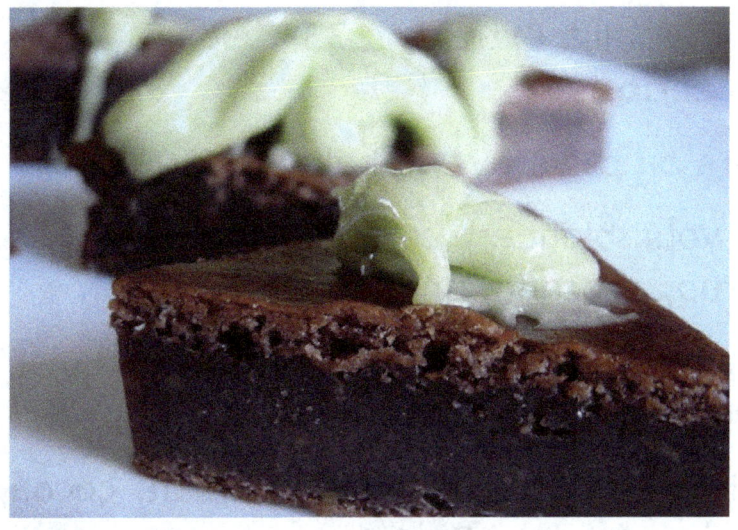

Preparation Time: 10 minutes.

Cooking Time: 30 minutes.

Servings: 16.

Ingredients:

- Ripe avocado – 1 Large.
- Organic eggs – 3 Large.
- Unsweetened apple sauce – .5 Cup.
- Sea salt – .25 Tsp.
- Coconut flour – .5 Cup.
- Maple syrup – .5 Cup.
- Baking soda – 1 Tsp.

- Unsweetened Dutch cocoa powder – .5 Cup.
- Vanilla extract – .33 Tbsp.

Directions:

Turn on the stove to bake at 350ºF.

In your blender, combine the vanilla, maple syrup, avocado, and apple sauce.

Move the ingredients to a large bowl, add eggs, and whisk together.

Stir in the coconut flour, sea salt, cocoa, and baking soda. Continue stirring until well combined.

Use coconut oil to grease an 8x8 baking pan and pour in the batter.

Allow baking in the oven for about 25 minutes.

Once the brownies have cooled for 20 minutes, cut into 16 pieces.

Store the brownies unrefrigerated in an airtight container for up to 2 days.

Nutrition:

Calories: 139.0.   **Carbs:** 15.7 g.

Fat: 8.3 g.   **Protein:** 3.0 g.

Super Salads Recipes

Chicken & Kale Salad

Preparation Time: 20 minutes.

Cooking Time: 18 minutes.

Servings: 4.

Ingredients:

For Chicken:
- 1 teaspoon dried thyme
- ½ teaspoon garlic powder
- ½ teaspoon onion powder
- ¼ teaspoon cayenne pepper
- ¼ teaspoon ground turmeric
- Salt and ground black pepper, as required
- 2 (7-ounce) boneless, skinless chicken breasts, pounded into ¾-inch thickness
- 1 tablespoon olive oil

For Salad:

- 6 cups fresh kale, tough ribs removed and chopped
- 2 cups carrots, peeled and cut into matchsticks
- ¼ cup walnuts

For Dressing:

- 1 small garlic clove, minced
- 2 tablespoons fresh lime juice
- 2 tablespoons extra-virgin olive oil
- 1 teaspoon raw honey
- ½ teaspoon Dijon mustard
- Salt and ground black pepper, as required

Directions:

Preheat your oven to 425 °F.

Line a baking dish with parchment paper.

For chicken: in a bowl, mix together the thyme, spices, salt and black pepper.

Drizzle the chicken breasts with oil and then rub with spice mixture generously.

Arrange the chicken breasts onto the prepared baking dish.

Bake for approximately 16 - 18 minutes.

Remove the baking dish from oven and transfer chicken breasts onto a cutting board for about 5 minutes.

For salad: place all ingredients in a salad bowl and mix.

For dressing: place all ingredients in another bowl and beat until well combined.

Cut each chicken breast into desired sized slices.

Place the salad onto each serving plate and top each with chicken slices.

Drizzle with dressing and serve.

Nutrition:

Calories: 330.

Fat: 18.9 g.

Carbs: 16.5 g.

Protein: 25.3 g.

Chicken & Berries Salad

Preparation Time: 20 minutes.

Cooking Time: 16 minutes.

Servings: 8.

Ingredients:

- 2 pounds boneless, skinless chicken breasts
- ½ cup olive oil
- ¼ cup fresh lemon juice
- 2 tablespoons maple syrup
- 1 garlic clove, minced
- Salt and ground black pepper, as required
- 2 cups fresh strawberries, hulled and sliced
- 2 cups fresh blueberries
- 10 cups fresh baby arugula

Directions:

For marinade: in a large bowl, add oil, lemon juice, Erythritol, garlic, salt and black pepper and beat until well combined.

In a large resealable plastic bag, place the chicken and ¾ cup of marinade.

Seal bag and shake to coat well.

Refrigerate overnight.

Cover the bowl of remaining marinade and refrigerate before serving.

Preheat the grill to medium heat. Grease the grill grate.

Remove the chicken from bag and discard the marinade.

Place the chicken onto grill grate and grill, covered for about 5 - 8 minutes per side.

Remove chicken from grill and cut into bite-sized pieces.

In a large bowl, add the chicken pieces, strawberries and spinach and mix.

Place the reserved marinade and toss to coat.

Serve immediately.

Nutrition:

Calories: 377.

Fat: 21.5 g.

Carbs: 12.6 g.

Protein: 34.1 g.

Chicken Salad

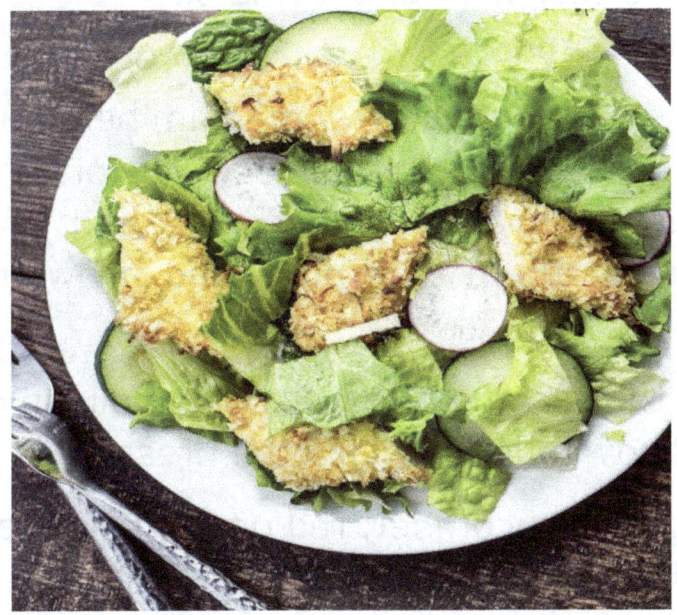

Preparation time: 5 Minutes.

Cooking Time: 30 Minutes.

Servings: 2.

Ingredients:

- ½ red onion, very finely sliced
- 1 tablespoon of sesame seeds
- 150g of cooked chicken-shredded
- Large handful 20g of parsley-chopped
- 100g of baby kale-chopped roughly
- 2 teaspoons of soy sauce

- 1 teaspoon of clear honey
- 1 teaspoon of sesame oil

Directions:

Place a frying pan over medium heat and toast the sesame seeds in the dry pan for 2 minutes until they are light brown and fragrant. Transfer them to a plate and allow them to cool.

Mix the sesame oil, honey, olive oil, lime juice, and soy sauce to make the dressing.

Place the cucumber, red onion, kale, pak choi, and parsley in a large bowl and gently mix. Pour the dressing over and mix again.

Split the salad into two plates and place the shredded chicken on top.

Just before serving, sprinkle the sesame seeds.

Nutrition:

Calories: 370.

Carbs: 1g.

Fat: 33g.

Protein: 14g.

Soups and Broths Recipes

Lentil Soup

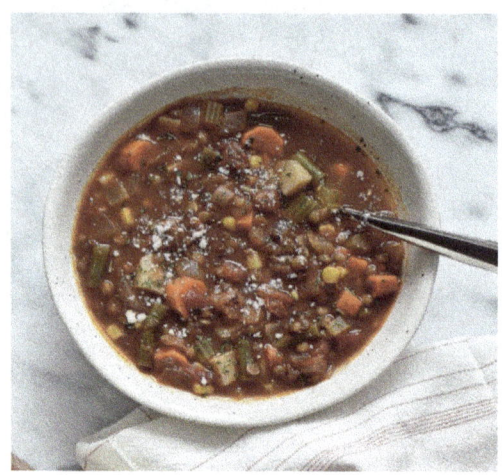

Preparation Time: 5 minutes.

Cooking Time: 1 hour and 5 minutes.

Servings: 4.

Ingredients:

- 175g (6oz) red lentils
- 1 red onion, chopped
- 1 clove of garlic, chopped
- 2 sticks of celery, chopped

- 2 carrots, chopped
- ½ bird's-eye chili
- 1 teaspoon ground cumin
- 1 teaspoon ground turmeric
- 1 teaspoon ground coriander (cilantro)
- 1200mls (2 pints) vegetable stock (broth)
- 2 tablespoons olive oil
- Sea salt
- Freshly ground black pepper

Directions:

Heat the oil in a saucepan and add the onion and cook for 5 minutes.

Add in the carrots, lentils, celery, chili, coriander (cilantro), cumin, turmeric and garlic and cook for 5 minutes.

Pour in the stock (broth), bring it to the boil, reduce the heat and simmer for 45 minutes.

Using a hand blender or food processor, puree the soup until smooth.

Season with salt and pepper. Serve.

Nutrition:

Calories: 94.   **Carbs:** 34g.

Fat: 1g.   **Protein:** 13g.

Spicy Pumpkin Soup

Preparation Time: 17 minutes.

Cooking Time: 28 minutes.

Servings: 4.

Ingredients:

- 150g (5oz) kale
- 1 butternut squash, peeled, de-seeded and chopped
- 1 red onion, chopped
- 3 bird's-eye chilies, chopped
- 3 cloves of garlic
- 2 teaspoons turmeric
- 1 teaspoon ground ginger
- 600mls (1 pint) vegetable stock (broth)
- 2 tablespoons olive oil

Directions:

Heat the olive oil in a saucepan, add the chopped butternut squash and onion and cook for 6 minutes until softened.

Stir in the kale, garlic, chili, turmeric and ginger and cook for 2 minutes, stirring constantly.

Pour in the vegetable stock (broth) bring it to the boil and cook for 20 minutes.

Using a food processor or a hand blender process until smooth.

Serve on its own or with a swirl of cream or crème fraiche. Enjoy.

Nutrition:

Calories: 164.8.

Fat: 4.3 g.

Carbs: 32g.

Protein: 22g.

Speedy Suppers Recipes

Kale and Turmeric Chicken Salad and Honey Lime Dressing

Preparation Time: 20 minutes.

Cooking Time: 10 minutes.

Servings: 2.

Ingredients:

For the Chicken:

- Chicken thighs – 9 oz./ 300 g (diced)
- Coconut oil – 1 tablespoon, or ghee – 1 teaspoon
- Turmeric powder – 1 teaspoon
- Medium brown onion – ½ (diced)
- Large garlic clove – 1 (finely chopped)
- Juice of a half lime
- Lime zest – 1 teaspoon
- Pepper and salt, to taste – ½ teaspoon

For the Salad:

- A handful of fresh parsley leaves – chopped
- A handful of fresh coriander leaves – chopped
- Kale – 3 large leaves (stems removed and leaves chopped)
- Pumpkin seeds – 2 tablespoons
- Broccoli florets – 2 cups, or broccoli stalks – 6
- Avocado – ½ (sliced)

For the Dressing:

- Raw honey – 1 teaspoon
- Lime juice – 3 tablespoons
- Pepper and sea salt, to taste – ½ teaspoon
- Dijon mustard or wholegrain – ½ teaspoon
- Small garlic clove – 1 (grated or finely diced)
- Extra-virgin olive oil – 3 tablespoons

Directions:

Get your chicken ready. Heat your coconut oil in a small fry-pan over medium-high heat. Add the chopped onion and sauté until golden, this will take about five minutes. Add the garlic and the diced chicken, stir for another two to three minutes to break it apart.

Add the lime juice and zest, turmeric powder, pepper, and salt and cook for another four minutes, stirring occasionally. Set aside once the time is up.

While cooking the chicken, add water to a small saucepan and allow to boil. Add the broccolini once the water is boiled and cook for approx. two minutes. Rinse the vegetable under cold water and cut into 3 or 4 pieces each.

Add the pumpkin seeds to a dry fry-pan and toast over medium heat for approx. two minutes, while occasionally stirring to prevent the seeds from getting burnt. Season with a little salt. Set aside. You may also use the pumpkin seeds raw if you want.

Add the chopped kale into your salad bowl and pour over your dressing. Use your fingers to massage and toss the kale with the dressing to soften the kale.

Now add the sliced avocado, pumpkin seeds, broccolini, cooked chicken, fresh parsley, and coriander leaves. Toss together. Serve.

Note: You may use chopped fish, prawn, or beef mince in place of the chicken.

Nutrition:

Calories: 229.

Fat: 27.6g.

Carbs: 30.3g.

Protein: 6.7g.

Turmeric Baked Salmon

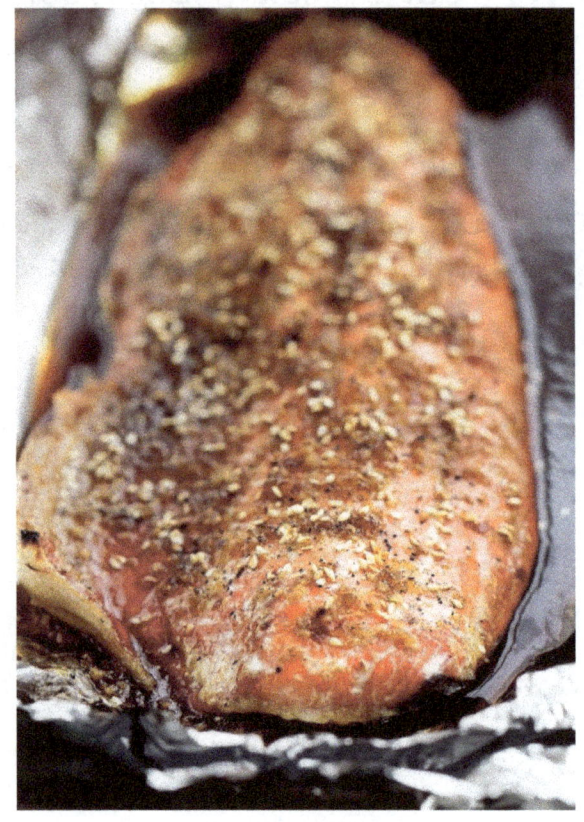

Preparation Time: 15 minutes.

Cooking Time: 10 minutes.

Servings: 1.

Ingredients:

- Skinned Salmon – 5 ounces
- ¼ juice of a lemon
- Ground turmeric - 1 teaspoon
- Extra virgin olive oil - 1 teaspoon

For the Spicy Celery:

- Chicken or vegetable stock - 100 ml
- Extra virgin olive oil - 1 teaspoon
- Chopped parsley - 1 tablespoon
- Tinned green lentils – ½ cup
- Red onion – 1/3 cup (finely chopped)
- Fresh ginger - 1 cm (finely chopped)
- Garlic clove – 1 (finely chopped)
- Bird's eye chili – 1 (finely chopped)
- Celery – 5 ounces (cut into 2cm lengths)
- Mild curry powder - 1 teaspoon
- Tomato – 4.6 ounces (cut into eight wedges)

Directions:

Heat your oven to 200°C or 390°F.

Begin with the spicy celery. Heat your frypan over medium-low heat, add the olive oil, and then add the onion, celery, ginger, garlic, and chili. Fry for about three minutes or until soft but not colored. Then add the curry powder and cook for another minute.

Add the tomatoes, stock, and lentils. Simmer gently for approx. ten minutes. Feel free to decrease or increase your cooking time, depending on how crunchy you like your celery.

Mix the lemon juice, oil, and turmeric in a small bowl. Rub the mixture over the salmon. Place on a baking tray and place in the oven to cook for about ten minutes.

Once done, stir the parsley through the celery and serve with the cooked salmon.

Nutrition:

Calories: 426.

Fat: 22g.

Carbs: 26g.

Protein: 26g.

Buckwheat with Chicken, Kale and Miso Dressing

Preparation Time: 15 minutes.

Cooking Time: 15 minutes.

Servings: 2.

Ingredients:

- Kales leaves – 3 handfuls (removed from the stem and chop roughly)
- Shiitake mushrooms – 4 (sliced)
- Tamari sauce (gluten-free soy sauce) – 3 tablespoons
- Brown onion – 1 (finely chopped)
- Buckwheat noodles – 5 oz. (100% buckwheat, no wheat)
- Ghee or coconut oil – 1 teaspoon
- Large garlic cloves – 2 (finely diced)
- Free-range chicken breast, medium size – 1 (washed and diced)
- Long red chili – 1 (thinly sliced, remove the seeds if you do not want it too hot)

For the Miso Dressing:

- Lime or lemon juice – 1 tablespoon
- Fresh organic miso – 1 ½ tablespoons
- Extra virgin olive oil – 1 tablespoon
- Tamari sauce – 1 tablespoon
- Sesame oil – 1 tablespoon (optional)

Directions:

Add water to a medium-sized pot and allow to boil. Add the kale and cook for approx. one minute or until slightly wilted. Take out the kale leaves and set aside while you reserve the water in the pot. Bring the water back to a boil, then add the soba noodles and cook following the instructions on the package. Rinse under cold water once cooked, then set aside.

While the noodle is getting ready, add one teaspoon of the coconut oil or ghee to a fry-pan, add the shiitake mushrooms once the oil is heated, then fry for approx. three minutes or until the mushrooms are lightly browned on each side. Sprinkle with sea salt, then set aside.

Using the same fry-pan, heat more ghee or coconut oil over medium-high heat. Add the onion and chili into the pan, sauté for about 2 minutes, then add the pieces of the chicken. Cook for another five minutes over medium heat, while stirring occasionally. Add the tamari sauce, garlic, and a little splash of water. Cook for another 3 minutes while occasionally stirring until the chicken is well cooked.

Now add the soba noodles and the kale to the pan and toss with the chicken to warm up.

Mix the miso dressing and sprinkle over the noodles once you are done cooking. This will ensure that the beneficial probiotics in the miso stay active and alive.

Nutrition:

Calories: 260.

Fat: 7g.

Carbs: 35g.

Protein: 15g.

Main Meals Recipe

Strawberry Buckwheat Tabbouleh

Preparation Time: 15 minutes.

Cooking Time: 10 minutes.

Servings: 2

Ingredients:

- 50g buckwheat
- 1 tablespoon turmeric
- 80g avocado
- 65g tomatoes
- 20 g red onion
- 25 g dates, pitted
- 1 tablespoon capers
- 30g parsley
- 100g strawberries
- 1 tablespoon of olive oil
- Juice of 1/2 lemon
- 30g rocket salad

Directions:

Boil the buckwheat together with turmeric and let it cool down.

Finely chop the avocado, tomatoes, red onions, dates, capers and parsley and mix with the cooled buckwheat. Cut the strawberries and mix with the rest—season with oil and lemon juice. Serve on the rocket.

Nutrition:

Calories: 141

Fat: 9.5 g.

Carbs: 13.4 g.

Protein: 2.8 g.

Chili Con Carne

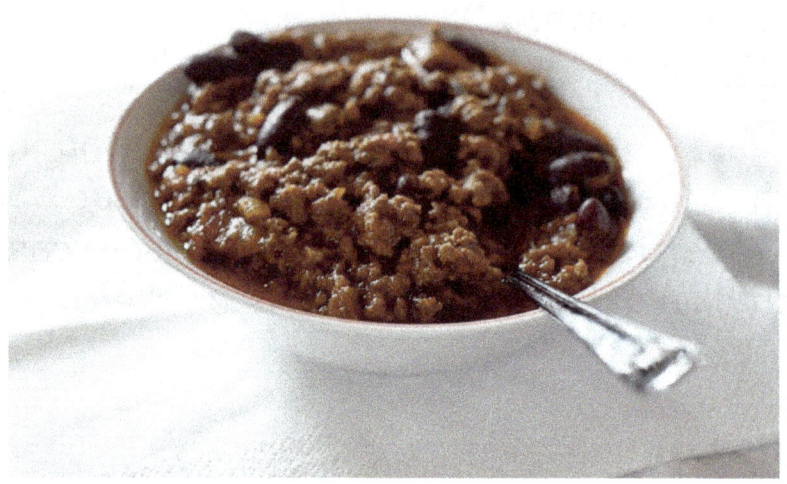

Preparation Time: 5 minutes.

Cooking Time: 30 minutes.

Servings: 3

Ingredients:

- 1 red onion, chopped
- 3 cloves of garlic, finely chopped
- 2 Tai chilies, finely chopped
- 1 tablespoon of olive oil
- 1 tablespoon turmeric
- 1 tablespoon cumin

- 400g minced beef
- 150ml red wine
- 1 red pepper, seeded and diced
- 2 cans of small tomatoes (400ml each)
- 1 tablespoon of tomato paste
- 1 tablespoon cocoa powder (without sugar)
- 150g canned kidney beans, drained
- 300ml beef broth
- 5g coriander green, chopped
- 5g parsley, chopped
- 160g buckwheat

Directions:

Sauté the onions, garlic and chilies in olive oil in a high frying pan or in a frying pan at medium heat. After three minutes, add cumin and turmeric and stir.

Then add the minced meat and fry until everything is brown. Add the red wine, bring to the boil and reduce by half.

Add the peppers, tomatoes, tomato paste, cocoa, kidney beans and stock, stir and cook for an hour. Add a little water or broth if the chili is too dry.

Cook buckwheat according to the instructions on the packet and serve sprinkled with the chilies and fresh herbs.

Nutrition:

Calories 292.2

Fat: 11.0 g.

Carbohydrate: 20.0 g.

Protein: 26.0 g.

Spinach and Eggplant Casserole

Preparation Time: 15 minutes.

Cooking Time: 55 minutes.

Servings: 3

Ingredients:

- Eggplant
- Onion slices
- A spoon of olive oil
- 450 g spinach (fresh)
- Tomato
- Egg
- 60 ml of almond milk
- 1 teaspoon lemon juice
- Almond flour

Directions:

Preheat the oven to 200 ° C.

Brush the eggplant and onions with olive oil and fry them in the pan.

Place spinach in a large pot, heat over medium heat, then drain the colander.

Put the vegetables in a frying pan: first eggplant, then spinach, then onions and tomatoes. Repeat again

Beat eggs with almond milk, lemon juice, salt and pepper, then pour them on the vegetables.

Sprinkle almond flour on a plate and bake for about 30 to 40 minutes.

Nutrition:

Calories: 139.9

Fat: 6.5 g.

Carbohydrate: 21.5 g.

Protein: 10.3 g.

Desserts Recipes

Green Tea and Vanilla Cream

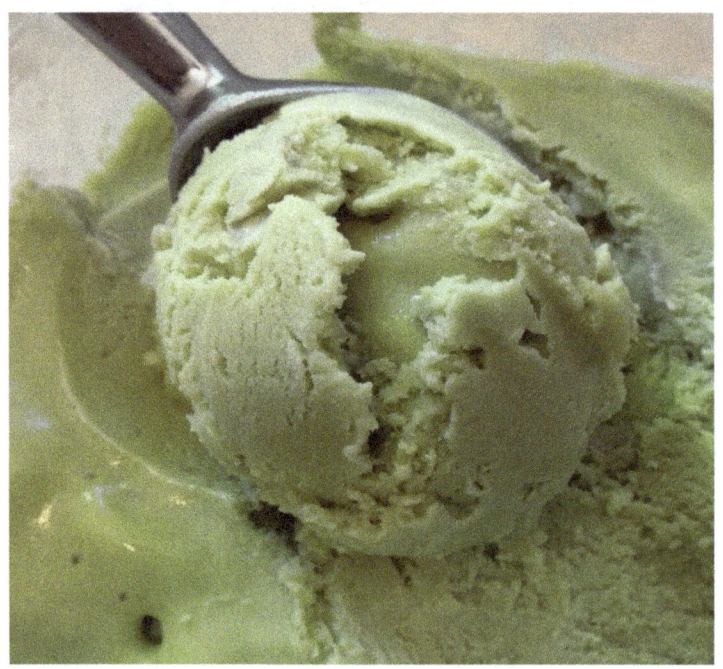

Preparation Time: 2 hours.

Cooking Time: 0 minutes.

Servings: 4

Ingredients:

- 14 ounces almond milk, hot
- 2 tablespoons green tea powder
- 14 ounces heavy cream
- 3 tablespoons stevia
- 1 teaspoon vanilla extract
- 1 teaspoon gelatin powder

Directions:

In a bowl, combine the almond milk with the green tea powder and the rest of the ingredients, whisk well, cool down, divide into cups and keep in the fridge for 2 hours before serving.

Nutrition:

Calories: 120

Fat: 3g.

Carbs: 7g.

Protein: 4g.

Figs Pie

Preparation Time: 10 minutes.

Cooking Time: 1 hour.

Servings: 8

Ingredients:

- ½ cup stevia
- 6 figs, cut into quarters
- ½ teaspoon vanilla extract
- 1 cup almond flour
- 4 eggs, whisked

Directions:

Spread the figs on the bottom of a springform pan lined with parchment paper.

In a bowl, combine the other ingredients, whisk and pour over the figs.

Bake at 375ºF for 1 hour, flip the pie upside down when it's done and serve.

Nutrition:

Calories: 200   **Carbs:** 7.6g.

Fat: 4.4g.   **Protein:** 8g.

Chocolate and Chili Tart

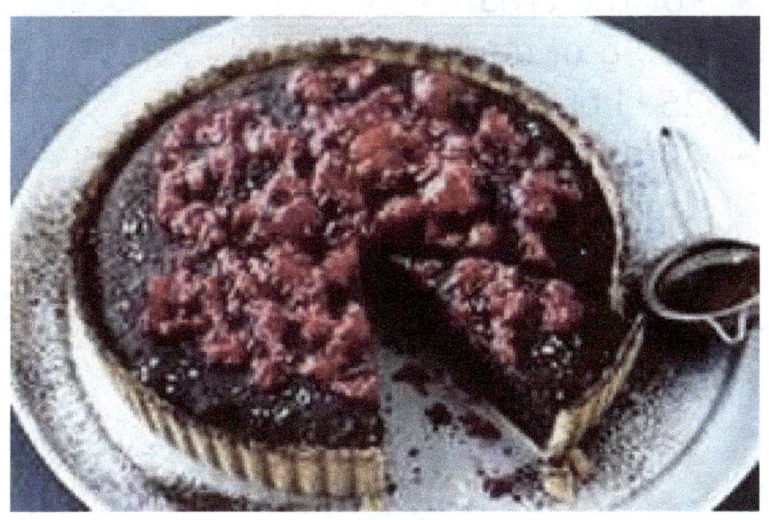

Preparation Time: 5 Minutes.

Cooking time: 25 Minutes.

Servings: 2

Ingredients:

For the mixture:
- 200 g of flour
- 100 g of butter
- 2 yolks
- 50 g of icing sugar

- 1 pinch of salt
- For the cream:
- 200 g of dark chocolate
- 25 cl of fresh cream
- 20 g of butter
- 1 pinch of hot pepper powder

To seal:

- Fresh red chilies
- 40 g of sugar

Directions:

Combine the flour with the icing sugar and a pinch of salt in the mixer, add the diced cold butter and whisk until a crumb mixture is formed. Add the yolks, blend again for a few seconds and wrap the pasta in a sheet of plastic wrap.

Roll out the pastry to 2 - 3 millimeters and line the greased mold. Remove the excess, pierce the bottom with a fork, cover the pasta with a wet and dried sheet of parchment paper, fill it with the appropriate weights and cook the base in white for about 15 minutes. Remove paper and weights and continue cooking for another 5 - 6 minutes.

Let the pasta cool, pour the prepared ganache and let the cake cool in the fridge for at least two hours. In the meantime, clean the chilies and remove the internal seeds and the stalk. Pour the sugar into a saucepan, add the same weight of water and bring to a boil. Add the chilies and cook them for 10 minutes, until they are transparent. Drain them from the syrup and let them dry on a wire rack. Decorate the cake to taste and serve.

Nutrition:

Calories: 134

Fat: 8g.

Carbs: 12g.

Protein: 1g.

Beverage Recipes

Berry and Beet Smoothie

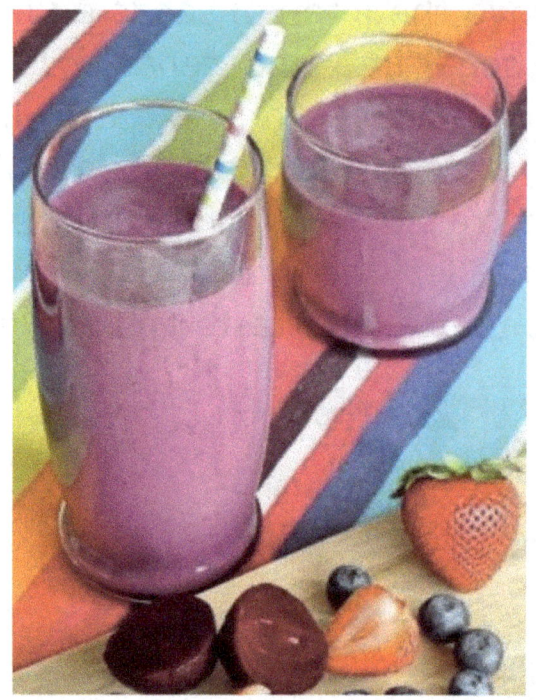

Preparation Time: 5 minutes.

Cooking Time: 0 minutes.

Servings: 2

Ingredients:

- 1 cup of pineapple juice
- 1 cup of low-fat or fat-free vanilla yogurt
- 1 cup of fresh or frozen strawberries
- 1/2 cup of fresh or frozen blueberries
- 1/2 cup of beet canned sliced, drained

Directions:

Combine all ingredients in a blender.

Mix until smooth.

Serve immediately.

Refrigerate or freeze what is left over during the next 2 hours.

Nutrition:

Calories: 166

Fat: 1g.

Carbohydrates: 40g.

Protein: 3g.

Irish Coffee

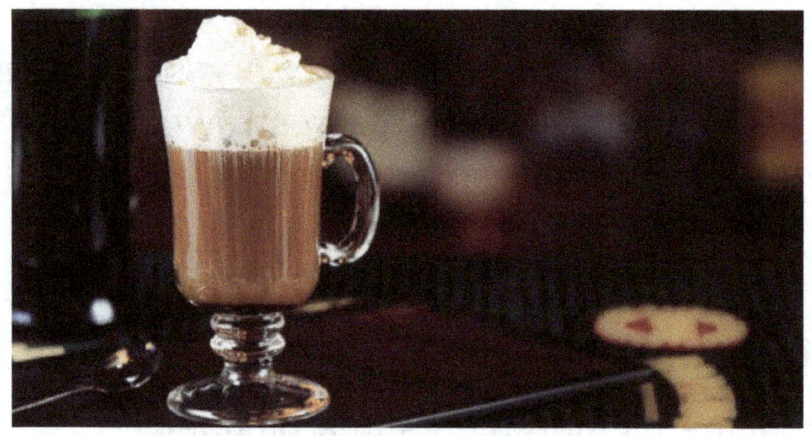

Preparation Time: 25 minutes.

Cooking Time: 0 minutes.

Servings: 1

Ingredients:

- 1.5 cl of cane sugar syrup (or 2 pieces of sugar)
- 2 cl of fresh cream
- 4 cl of coffee
- 3 cl of whiskey (bourbon, whiskey)

Directions:

Step 1

Make the "Irish Coffee" recipe directly in the glass.

2nd step

Heat the whiskey with the sugar (at low heat so as not to boil the whiskey) in a saucepan stirring. Prepare a black coffee and pour it over the hot and sweet whiskey, stir slightly. Pour everything into the rinsed glass with warm water and coat the surface with lightly beaten cream, it's ready! Savor without delay. To make your cream work better, place it in the freezer for 20 minutes before vigorously whipping it.

Despite some rumors of modern times, an Irish coffee is not supposed to have the three separate floors. Other variants can be made with whipped cream instead of fresh cream, liquid cane sugar instead of powdered sugar or replace the traditional whiskey with whiskey or bourbon, but the original recipe is the one explained above.

Step 3

Serve in a glass type "mug."

Step 4

Add any grated chocolate to the cream.

Nutrition:

Calories: 54

Fat: 4g.

Carbs: 6g.

Protein: 1g.

Double Melon Mojito

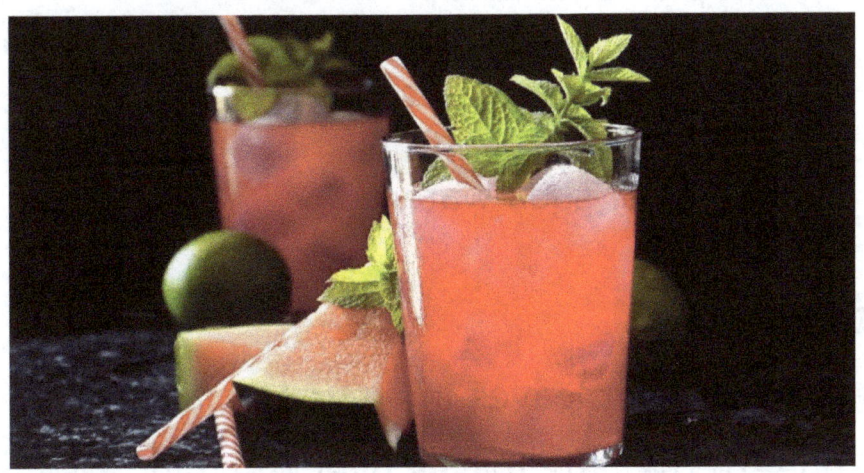

Preparation Time: 5 minutes.

Cooking Time: 0 minutes.

Servings: 1

Ingredients:

- 6 to 10 fresh mint leaves, plus 1 sprig to decorate
- 1 small file, cut in half, plus a slice to decorate
- ¼ cup melon in pieces (use any type, such as cantaloupe, Chinese melon or watermelon), plus some small pieces to garnish

- 2 tablespoons of simple stevia syrup or simple sugar syrup
- 1 line (1½ ounces) of white rum or rum flavored with melon
- 1 cup of ice
- ½ cup of soda water

Directions:

Place the mint leaves in a strong glass.

Squeeze the lime halves over the mint. Use a crusher to crush the mint and extract the aromatic oils lightly.

Add the melon and lightly squeeze it with the crusher.

Pour the syrup and rum into the glass, stirring. Stretch the preparation, if you prefer.

Add ice and soda water. Stir.

Dress the glass with the sprig of mint, the slice of the lime and the small pieces of melon, and let the melon pieces float in the drink.

Nutrition:

Calories: 96   **Carbs:** 13g.

Fat: 0.5g.   **Protein:** 11g.

Dinner Recipes

Blue Cheese Pork Chops

Preparation Time: 5 minutes.

Cooking Time: 10 minutes.

Servings: 2

Ingredients:

- 2 boneless pork chops
- Pink Himalayan salt
- Freshly ground black pepper
- 2 tablespoons butter
- ⅓ cup blue cheese crumbles
- ⅓ cup heavy (whipping) cream
- ⅓ cup sour cream

Directions:

Pat the pork chops dry, and season with pink Himalayan salt and pepper.

In a medium skillet over medium heat, melt the butter. When the butter melts and is very hot, add the pork chops and sear on each side for 3 minutes.

Transfer the pork chops to a plate and let rest for 3 to 5 minutes.

In a medium saucepan over medium heat, melt the blue cheese crumbles, stirring frequently, so they don't burn.

Add the cream and the sour cream to the pan with the blue cheese. Let simmer for a few minutes, stirring occasionally.

For an extra kick of flavor in the sauce, pour the pork-chop pan juice into the cheese mixture and stir. Let simmer while the pork chops are resting.

Put the pork chops on two plates, pour the blue cheese sauce over the top of each, and serve.

Nutrition:

Calories: 669

Fat: 34g.

Carbs: 4g.

Protein: 41g.

Carnitas

Preparation Time: 10 minutes.

Cooking Time: 8 hours.

Servings: 2

Ingredients:

- ½ tablespoon chili powder
- 1 tablespoon olive oil
- 1-pound boneless pork butt roast
- 2 garlic cloves, minced
- ½ small onion, diced
- Pinch pink Himalayan salt
- Pinch freshly ground black pepper
- Juice of 1 lime

Directions:

With the crock insert in place, preheat the slow cooker to low.

In a small bowl, mix to combine the chili powder and olive oil, and rub it all over the pork.

Place the pork in the slow cooker, fat-side up.

Top the pork with the garlic, onion, pink Himalayan salt, pepper, and lime juice.

Cover and cook on low for 8 hours.

Transfer the pork to a cutting board, shred the meat with two forks, and serve.

Nutrition:

Calories: 446

Fat: 26g.

Carbs: 4g.

Protein: 45g.

Carnitas Nachos

Preparation Time: 5 minutes

Cooking Time: 10 minutes

Servings: 2

Ingredients:

- 1 tablespoon olive oil, plus more for coating
- 2 cups pork rinds (I use spicy flavor)
- ½ cup shredded cheese (I use Mexican blend)
- 1 cup Carnitas
- 1 avocado, diced
- 2 tablespoons sour cream

Directions:

Preheat the oven to 350°F. Coat a 9 – by – 13 - inch baking dish with olive oil.

Put the pork rinds in the prepared baking dish, and top with the cheese.

Put in the oven and bake until the cheese has melted about 5 minutes. Transfer to a cooling rack and let rest for 5 minutes.

In a medium skillet over high heat, heat the olive oil. Put the carnitas in the skillet, and add some of the reserved pan juices. Cook for a few minutes, until you get a nice crispy crust on the carnitas, and then flip the carnitas to the other side and cook briefly.

Divide the heated pork rinds and cheese between two plates.

Top the pork rinds and cheese with the reheated carnitas, add the diced avocado and a dollop of sour cream to each, and serve hot.

Nutrition:

Calories: 587

Fat: 51g.

Carbs: 5g.

Protein: 51g.

Other Sirtfood Recipes

Turkey Breakfast Sausages

Preparation Time:

Cooking Time:

Servings:

Ingredients:

- 1 lb. extra lean ground turkey
- 1 Tbsp. EVOO, and a little more to dirt pan
- 1 Tbsp. fennel seeds
- 2 teaspoons smoked paprika
- 1 teaspoon red pepper flakes
- 1 teaspoon peppermint
- 1 teaspoon chicken seasoning
- A couple of shredded cheddar cheese
- A couple of chives, finely chopped
- A few shakes garlic and onion powder
- Two spins of pepper and salt

Directions:

Pre Heat oven to 350ºF.

Utilize a little EVOO to dirt a miniature muffin pan.

Combine all Ingredients: and blend thoroughly.

Fill each pit on top of the pan and then cook for approximately 15 - 20 minutes. Each toaster differs; therefore, when muffin fever is 165, then remove.

Nutrition:

Calories: 70.

Fat: 3.5 g.

Carbohydrates: 0 g.

Protein: 2g.

Banana and Blueberry Muffins

Preparation Time: 10 minutes.

Cooking Time: 20 minutes.

Servings: 12

Ingredients:

- 4 large ripe bananas, peeled and mashed
- 3/4 cup of sugar
- 1 egg, lightly crushed
- 1/2 cup of butter, melted (and a little extra to dust the interiors of this muffin tin)
- 2 cups of blueberries (if they are suspended, do not Defrost them. simply pop them into the batter suspended and)
- 1 teaspoon baking powder
- 1 teaspoon baking soda
- 1/2 teaspoon salt
- 1 cup of coconut bread
- 1/2 cup of flour (or 1 - 1; two cup bread)
- 1/2 cup applesauce
- Dab of cinnamon

Directions:

Add mashed banana to a large mixing bowl.

Insert sugar & egg and mix well.

Add peanut butter and strawberries.

Sift all the dry Ingredients together, then add the dry Ingredients: into the wet mix and mix together lightly.

Set into 12 greased muffin

Bake for 20 - 30min in 180ºC or 350ºF.

Nutrition:

Calories: 229.6

Fat: 9.5g.

Carbs: 8.3g.

Protein: 4.2g.

Morning Meal Sausage Gravy

Preparation Time: 5 minutes.

Cooking Time: 10 minutes.

Servings: 8

Ingredients:

- 1 lb. sausage
- 2 cups 2 percent milk (complete is great also)
- 1/4 cup entire wheat bread
- Salt and a Lot of pepper to flavor

Directions:

Cook sausage from skillet.

Add flour and blend cook for about a minute.

Insert two cups of milk.

Whisk whilst gravy thickens and bubbles.

Add pepper and salt and keep to taste until flawless.

Let stand a minute or so to ditch and function over several snacks.

Nutrition:

Calories: 361.8

Fat: 17.0g.

Carbs: 14.0g.

Protein: 11.2g.

CONCLUSION

Congratulations on making it to the end of this book. The Sirtfood diet promotes solid foods, however it is prohibitive in calorie and nutrition decisions. It also includes drinking bunches of juice, which is far from a valid suggestion. Despite the fact that the main period of the Sirtfood diet is exceptionally low in calories and healthily inadequate, there are no real wellness concerns for the normal, healthy adult who thinks about the short-term diet. However, for someone with diabetes, calorie restriction and alcohol consumption typically squeezing for the first few days of the diet can cause risky changes in glucose levels.

In any case, even a healthy individual may encounter some reactions, mainly hunger. I hope my recipes and meal plan have changed your lifestyle and helped you achieve your goal. Good luck.

CPSIA information can be obtained
at www.ICGtesting.com
Printed in the USA
BVHW090756260521
607981BV00010B/34